The Essential Sirt Food Diet Recipe

A Quick Start Guide To Cooking on The Sirt Food Diet

2

Sommario

INTRODUCTION

Of the hundreds of millions of people adopting popular diets this year, less than 1% will achieve significant weight loss. Not only are they failing to make a difference in the war of the bulge, they are doing nothing to stem the tide of chronic disease that has swept through modern society.

That's why I decided to write this book, to delight you with recipes that are healthy, light, but also very tasty and full of nutrition and flavor.

Your family will thank you for letting them try these dishes, but let's not waste time, put on your apron, prepare the kitchen we start cooking.

BREAKFAST RECIPES

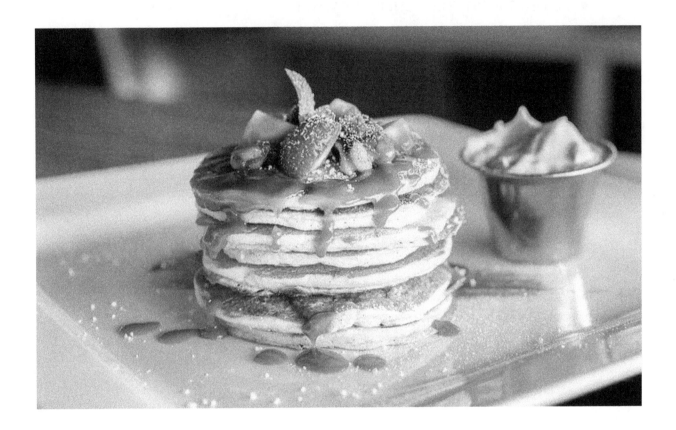

Mushroom Scramble Eggs

Ingredients

- 2 tbsp

- 1 teaspoon ground garlic

- 1 teaspoon mild curry powder

- 20g lettuce, approximately sliced

- 1 teaspoon extra virgin olive oil

- 1/2 bird's eye peeled, thinly chopped

- a couple of mushrooms, finely chopped

- 5g parsley, finely chopped

- *elective * Insert a seed mix for a topper plus Some Rooster Sauce for taste

Guidelines

- Mix the curry and garlic powder and then add just a little water till you've achieved a light glue.

- Steam the lettuce for two -- 3 minutes.

- Heat the oil in a skillet over a moderate heat and fry the chili and mushrooms 2-- three minutes till they've begun to soften and brown.

- Insert the eggs and spice paste and cook over moderate heat, then add the carrot and then proceed to cook over a moderate heat for a further minute. In the end, put in the parsley, mix well, and function.

Blue Hawaii Smoothie

Ingredients

- 2 tablespoons rings or approximately 4-5 balls

- 1/2 cup frozen tomatoes

- two Tbsp ground flaxseed

- ⅛ cup tender coconut (unsweetened, organic)

- few walnuts

- 1/2 cup fat-free yogurt

- 5-6 ice cubes

- dab of water

Guidelines

- Throw all of the **Ingredients** together and combine until smooth. You might need to prevent and wake up to receive it combined smoothy or put in more water.

Turkey Breakfast Sausages

Ingredients

- 1 lb extra lean ground turkey

- 1 Tbsp EVOO, and a little more to dirt pan

- 1 Tbsp fennel seeds

- 2 teaspoon smoked paprika

- 1 teaspoon red pepper flakes

- 1 teaspoon peppermint

- 1 teaspoon chicken seasoning

- A couple of shredded cheddar cheese

- A couple of chives, finely chopped

- A few shakes garlic and onion powder

- Two spins of pepper and salt

Guidelines

- Pre Heat oven to 350F.

- Utilize a little EVOO to dirt a miniature muffin pan.

- Combine all **Ingredients** and blend thoroughly.

- Fill each pit on top of the pan and then cook for approximately 15-20 minutes. Each toaster differs; therefore, when muffin fever is 165, then remove.

Banana Pecan Muffins

Ingredients

- 3 Tbsp butter softened

- 4 ripe bananas

- 1 Tbsp honey

- ⅛ cup OJ

- 1 teaspoon cinnamon

- 2 cups all-purpose pasta

- 2 capsules

- a couple of pecans, sliced

- 1 Tbsp vanilla

Guidelines

- Preheat the oven to 180ºC/ / 350ºF.

- Lightly grease the bottom and sides of the muffin tin, and then dust with flour.

- Dust the surfaces of the tin gently with flour then tap to eradicate any excess.

- Peel and insert the batter to a mixing bowl and with a fork, mash the carrots; therefore that you've got a combination of chunky and smooth, then put aside.

- Insert the orange juice, melted butter, eggs, vanilla, and spices and stir to combine.

- Roughly chop the pecans onto a chopping board, when using, then fold throughout the mix.

- Spoon at the batter 3/4 full and bake in the oven for approximately 40 minutes, or until golden and cooked through.

Banana And Blueberry Muffins - SRC

Ingredients

- 4 large ripe banana, peeled and mashed

- 3/4 cup of sugar

- 1 egg, lightly crushed

- 1/2 cup of butter, melted (and a little extra to dust the interiors of this muffin tin)

- 2 cups of blueberries (if they are suspended, do not defrost them. simply pop them into the batter suspended and)

- 1 teaspoon baking powder

- 1 teaspoon baking soda

- 1/2 teaspoon salt

- 1 cup of coconut bread

- 1/2 cup of flour (or 1-1;two cup bread)

- 1/2 cup applesauce

- dab of cinnamon

Guidelines

- Add mashed banana to a large mixing bowl.

- Insert sugar & egg and mix well.

- Add peanut butter and strawberries.

- Sift all the dry **Ingredients** together, then add the dry **Ingredients** into the wet mix and mix together lightly.

- Set into 12 greased muffin cups

- Bake for 20-30min in 180C or 350 F.

Morning Meal Sausage Gravy

Ingredients

- 1 lb sausage

- 2 cups 2 percent milk (complete is great also)

- 1/4 cup entire wheat bread

- salt and a Lot of pepper to flavor

Guidelines

- Cook sausage from skillet.

- Add flour and blend cook for about a minute.

- Insert two cups of milk.

- Whisk Whilst gravy thickens and bubbles.

- Add pepper and salt and keep to taste until flawless.

- Let stand a minute or so to ditch and function over several snacks.

Easy Egg-white Muffins

Ingredients

- Language muffin - I enjoy Ezekiel 7 grain

- egg-whites - 6 tbsp or two large egg whites

- turkey bacon or bacon sausage

- sharp cheddar cheese or gouda

- green berry

- discretionary - lettuce, and hot sauce, hummus, flaxseeds, etc.

Guidelines

- At a microwavable safe container, then spray entirely to stop the egg from adhering, then pour egg whites into the dish.

- Lay turkey bacon or bacon sausage paper towel and then cook .

- Subsequently, toast your muffin, if preferred.

- Then put the egg dish in the microwave for 30 minutes. Afterward, with a spoon or fork, then immediately flip egg within the dish and cook for another 30 minutes.

- Whilst dish remains hot sprinkle some cheese while preparing sausage.

- The secret is to get a paste of some kind between each coating to put up the sandwich together, i.e., a very small little bit of hummus or even cheese.

Sweet Potato Hash

Ingredients

- 1 Sweet-potato

- 1/2 red pepper, diced

- 3 green onions, peppermint

- leftover turkey, then sliced into bits (optional)

- 1 Tbsp of butter - perhaps a bit less (I never quantify)

- carrot powder - a few shakes

- Pepper - only a small dab to get a bit of warmth

- pepper and salt to flavor

- scatter of cheddar cheese (optional)

Guidelines

- Stab a sweet potato and microwave for 5 minutes.

- Remove from microwave, peel the skin off, and foliage.

- At a skillet, on medium-high warmth, place peppers and butter and sauté to get a few minutes.

- Insert potato bits and keep sautéing.

- Whilst sauté, add sweeteners, leafy vegetables, and green onions.

- Insert a dab of cheddar and Revel in!

Asparagus, Mushroom Artichoke Strata

Ingredients

- 1 little loaf of sourdough bread

- 4 challah rolls

- 8 eggs

- 2 cups of milk

- 1 teaspoon salt

- 1/4 teaspoon black pepper

- 1 cup Fontina cheese, cut into little chunks

- 1/2 cup shredded Parmesan cheese

- 1 Tbsp butter (I used jojoba)

- 1 teaspoon dried mustard

- 1/2 can of artichoke hearts, sliced

- 1 bunch green onions, grated

- 1 bunch asparagus, cut into 1-inch bits

- 1 10oz package of baby Bella (cremini) mushrooms, chopped

Guidelines

1. Clean mushrooms and slice and trim asparagus and cut in 1-inch pieces. Reserve in a bowl and scatter 1/2 teaspoon salt mixture.

2. Drain and dice 1/2 may or modest artichoke hearts.

3. Melt butter in a pan over moderate heat, also sauté the asparagus and mushrooms before the mushrooms start to brown, about 10 minutes.

4. Blend the artichoke core pieces into a bowl with all a mushroom/asparagus mix. Setaside.

5. Cut or split a tiny sourdough loaf into 1-inch bits. (My loaf was a little too small, therefore that I used 4 challah rolls too)

6. Grease a 9x13 inch baking dish and generate a base coating of bread at the dish. Spread 1/2 cup of Fontina cheese bread, at a coating, and disperse half an apple mixture on the cheese.

7. Lay-down a different layer of these vegetables and bread and high using a 1/2 cup of Fontina cheese.

8. Whisk together eggs, salt, milk, dry mustard, and pepper into a bowl and then pour the egg mixture on the vegetables and bread.

9. Cover the dish, and then simmer for 3 weeks.

10.   Pre Heat oven to 375 degrees.

11.   Eliminate the casserole from the fridge and let stand for half an hour.

12.   Spread All the Parmesan cheese at a coating within the strata.

13.   Bake in the preheated oven until a knife inserted near the border comes out clean, 40 to 45 minutes. Let stand 5 to 10 minutes before cutting into squares.

Egg White Veggie Wontons w/Fontina topped w/ crispy Prosciutto

Ingredients

- 1 cup egg whites

- butter

- fontina cheese

- mixed shredded cheddar cheese

- broccoli I utilized wheat, chopped bits

- tomatoes - diced

- salt and pepper

- prosciutto - two pieces

Guidelines

1. Remove Won Ton wrappers out of the freezer.

2. Pre Heat oven to 350.

3. Spray miniature cupcake tin with cooking spray.

4. After wrappers begin to defrost, peel off them carefully - apart, one at a time and press cupcake tin lightly.

5. I sliced the wrappers having a little bit of peanut butter. (optional)

6. set a chunk of cheese in every bottom.

7. Satisfy desired lettuce - I used pre-cooked broccoli bits and diced tomatoes.

8. Pour egg whites all toppings.

9. Sprinkle each with some of those shredded cheddar cheese.

10.   Cook for approximately 15 minutes, but get started watching them afterward 10 - whenever they poof up - assess them poking the middle with a fork.

11.   While eggs are cooking, then spray a sheet of foil with cooking spray and then put 2 pieces of prosciutto onto it and then cook at exactly the exact same period as the egg whites. After 8 minutes, then take and let sit once it cools it becomes crispy and chop and high eggs!

Crunchy and Chewy Granola

Ingredients

- Two 1/4 cup old-style yogurt

- 1 Tbsp flax seeds

- 1/4 tsp kosher salt

- 1/2 tsp cinnamon

- 1/4 ground ginger

- 1/2 cup honey

- two Tbsp packaged splendid brown-sugar

- 3/4 cup ounces raw peppers

- 1/2 cup sliced peppers

- 1/2 cup golden raisins

- 1/2 cup dried cranberries

- 1 Tbsp vanilla sugar to earn put a used vanilla bean in a full bowl of sugar and allow simmer for per month at icebox.

Guidelines

1. Pre Heat oven to 300.

2. Line baking sheet with parchment paper.

3. Mix 9 components together.

4. Insert 1 cup hot tap water, then mix together with hands and spread into a thin coating over a baking sheet.

5. Bake for 60 minutes, stirring 2-3 days, before turning black gold brown.

6. Remove from the oven and let cool.

7. Stir in dried fruit.

8. Dust with sugar.

Blueberry Pancakes

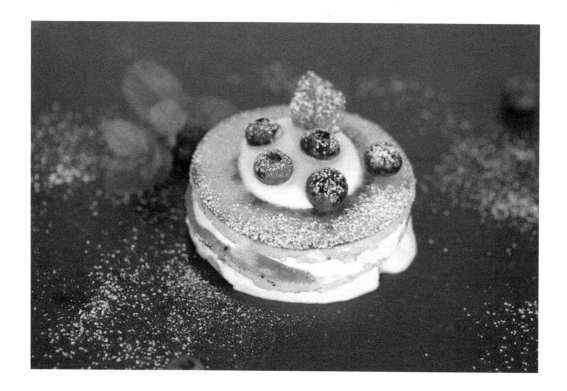

Ingredients

- 2 capsules

- 1 cup milk - then I used margarine

- 1 Tbsp vegetable oil

- 1.5 tsp butter melted, (and an additional piece of peanut butter to the pan)

- 1 1/4 cup All-purpose flour 3 tsp baking powder

- 3 tsp sugar

- 1/2 tsp salt

- 2 cups frozen blueberries

Guidelines

1. Put a nonstick griddle or a skillet over moderate heat.

2. Independent eggs yolks and whites, moving whites to some medium mixing bowl.

3. Whisk functions well with milk, butter, and oil.

4. Gradually fold dry **Ingredients** to liquid with a wooden spoon.

5. In yet another bowl, sift together dry skin.

6. Working with an electric beater, whip egg whites until frothy.

7. Pour egg whites into the batter until just combined (small bumps of eggwhite are fine).

8. When skillet is hot, brush the skillet with melted butter.

9. Pour 1/4 cup batter onto the skillet for each pancake, leaving space .

10.   Top each pancake using 5 6 blueberries, even if using.

11.   When bubbles form inside the batter, then flip the pancake.

12.   Keep on cooking until golden at the ground, about two minutes.

13.   Drink instantly.

Power Balls

Ingredients

- 1 cup old fashion ginger, dried (I've used apple cinnamon-flavored oats also)

- 1/4 cup quinoa cooked using 3/4 cup orange juice

- 1/4 cup shredded unsweetened coconut

- 1/3 cup dried cranberry/raisin blend

- 1/3 cup dark chocolate chips

- 1/4 cup slivered almonds

- 1 Tbsp reduced-fat peanut butter

Guidelines

1. Cook quinoa in orange juice. Bring to boil and simmer for approximately 1-2 minutes. Let cool.

2. Combine chilled quinoa and the remaining **Ingredients** into a bowl.

3. With wet hands and combine **Ingredients** and roll in golden ball sized chunks.

4. Set at a Tupperware and set in the refrigerator for two weeks until the firm.

Cinnamon Crescent Rolls

Ingredients

- 2 cans refrigerated crescent rolls

- 1 stick butter, softened

- 1/2 cup brown or white sugar

- 1 tbsp cinnamon

- Glaze

- 1/2 cup powdered sugar

- 1 tsp vanilla

- 2 tbsp milk

Guidelines

1. Heat oven to 350°F.

2. In a small bowl, combine sugar, butter, and cinnamon; beat until smooth.

3. Separate dough into rectangles.

4. Spread each rectangle about two tbsp cinnamon butter mix.

5. Roll-up starting at the broadest side, as you'll ordinarily do to crescent rolls. Firmly press ends to seal.

6. Put each cinnamon filled crescent roll on a parchment lineup baking sheet. *Be sure that you line the cookie sheet, or that you might have a large mess after *

7. Bake for 10 to 15 minutes or until golden brown.

8. In a small bowl, combine all glaze **Ingredients**, adding enough milk for desired drizzling consistency. Drizzle over hot rolls.

Fresh fruit Pizza

Ingredients

- 4 crescent rolls (Rolled-out and poked with a fork)

- Two spoonfuls of moderate Cream-cheese

- 1 teaspoon of sugar

- 1 teaspoon Vanilla extract

- Handful berries - chopped (You Can easily utilize lemon or blueberries)

- Sliced almonds

Guidelines

1. Place crescent rolls nonstick pan and then poke a few times with a fork. Cook at 375 for approximately 14 minutes. Let cool.

2. At a bowl, combine cream , Vanilla infusion & sugar stir with a spoon.

3. Spread onto crescent rolls, then add almonds and fruit.

4. I sprinkled a bit more sugar at the top after!

LUNCH RECIPES

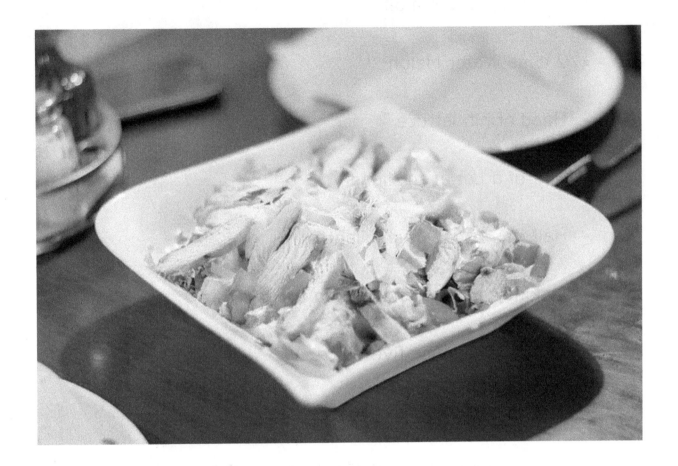

Sticky Chicken Water Melon Noodle Salad

Ingredients

- 2 pieces of skinny rice noodles

- 1/2 Tbsp sesame oil

- 2 cups Water Melon

- Head of bib lettuce

- Half of a Lot of scallions

- Half of a Lot of fresh cilantro

- 2 skinless, boneless chicken breasts

- 1/2 Tbsp Chinese five-spice

- 1 Tbsp extra virgin olive oil

- two Tbsp sweet skillet (I utilized a mixture of maple syrup using a dash of Tabasco)

- 1 Tbsp sesame seeds

- a couple of cashews - smashed

- Dressing - could be made daily or 2 until

- 1 Tbsp low-salt soy sauce

- 1 teaspoon sesame oil

- 1 Tbsp peanut butter

- Half of a refreshing red chili

- Half of a couple of chives

- Half of a couple of cilantro

- 1 lime - juiced

- 1 small spoonful of garlic

Guidelines

1. At a bowl, then completely substituting the noodles in boiling drinking water. They are going to soon be carried out in 2 minutes.

2. On a big sheet of parchment paper, then throw the chicken with pepper, salt, and also the five-spice.

3. Twist over the newspaper, subsequently celebration and put the chicken using a rolling pin.

4. Place into the large skillet with 1 Tbsp of olive oil, turning 3 or 4 minutes, until well charred and cooked through.

5. Drain the noodles and toss with 1 Tbsp of sesame oil onto a sizable serving dish.

6. Place 50% the noodles into the moderate skillet, stirring frequently until crispy and nice.

7. Eliminate the Watermelon skin, then slice the flesh to inconsistent balls and then increase the platter.

8. Reduce the lettuces and cut into small wedges and also half of a whole lot of leafy greens and scatter the dish.

9. Place another 1 / 2 the cilantro pack, the soy sauce, coriander, chives, peanut butter, and a dab of water, 1 teaspoon of sesame oil and the lime juice, then mix till smooth.

10. Set the chicken back to heat, garnish with all the sweet skillet (or my walnut syrup mixture), and toss with the sesame seeds.

11. Pour the dressing on the salad toss gently with fresh fingers until well coated, then add crispy noodles and then smashed cashews.

12.   Blend chicken pieces and add them to the salad.

Fruity Curry Chicken Salad

Ingredients

- 4 skinless, boneless Chicken Pliers - cooked and diced

- 1 tsp celery, diced

- 4 green onions, sliced

- 1 Golden Delicious apple peeled, cored and diced

- 1/3 cup golden raisins

- 1/3 cup seedless green grapes, halved

- 1/2 cup sliced toasted pecans

- ⅛ teaspoon ground black pepper

- 1/2 tsp curry powder

- 3/4 cup light mayonnaise

Instructions

• Measure 1

A big bowl, combine the chicken, onion, celery, apple, celery, celery, pecans, pepper, curry powder, and carrot. Mix altogether. Drink!

Turmeric Chicken & Kale Salad With Honey Lime Dressing- Sirtfood Recipes

Notes: When planning beforehand, dress the salad 10 minutes before serving. The chicken might be substituted with beef chopped, sliced prawns, or fish. Vegetarians may use chopped mushrooms or cooked quinoa.

Ingredients

For your poultry

* 1 tsp ghee or 1 tablespoon coconut oil

* 1/2 moderate brown onion, diced

* 250 300 grams / 9 oz. Chicken mince or pops upward Chicken thighs

* 1 large garlic clove, finely-manicured

* 1 tsp turmeric powder

* 1teaspoon lime zest

* juice of 1/2 lime

* 1/2 tsp salt

For your salad

* 6 broccolini 2 or two cups of broccoli florets

* two tbsp pumpkin seeds (pepitas)

* 3 big kale leaves, stalks removed and sliced

*1/2 avocado, chopped

* bunch of coriander leaves, chopped

* couple of fresh parsley leaves, chopped

For your dressing table

* 3 tbsp lime juice

* 1 small garlic clove, finely diced or grated

* 3 tbsp Extra-virgin Coconut Oil (I used 1. Tsp avocado oil and 2 tbsp EVO)

*1 tsp raw honey

* 1/2 tsp Whole Grain or Dijon mustard

* 1/2 tsp sea salt and salt

Guidelines

1. Heat the ghee or coconut oil at a Tiny skillet Pan above medium-high heat. Bring the onion and then sauté on moderate heat for 45 minutes, until golden. Insert the chicken blossom and garlic and simmer for 2-3 minutes on medium-high heat, breaking it all out.

2. Add the garlic, lime zest, lime juice, and salt and Soda and cook stirring often, to get a further 3-4 minutes. Place the cooked mince aside.

3. As the chicken is cooking, make a little Spoonful of water . Insert the broccolini and cook 2 minutes. Rinse under warm water and then cut into 3-4 pieces each.

4. Insert the pumpkin seeds into the skillet out of the Toast and chicken over moderate heat for two minutes, stirring often to avoid burning. Season with a little salt. Setaside. Raw pumpkin seeds will also be nice to utilize.

5. Put chopped spinach at a salad bowl and then pour over The dressing table. With the hands, massage, and toss the carrot with the dressing table. This will dampen the lettuce, a lot similar to what citrus juice will not steak or fish carpaccio – it 'hamburgers' it marginally.

6. Finally, throw throughout the cooked chicken, Broccolini, fresh herbs, pumpkin seeds, and avocado pieces.

Lamb, Butternut Squash And Date Tagine

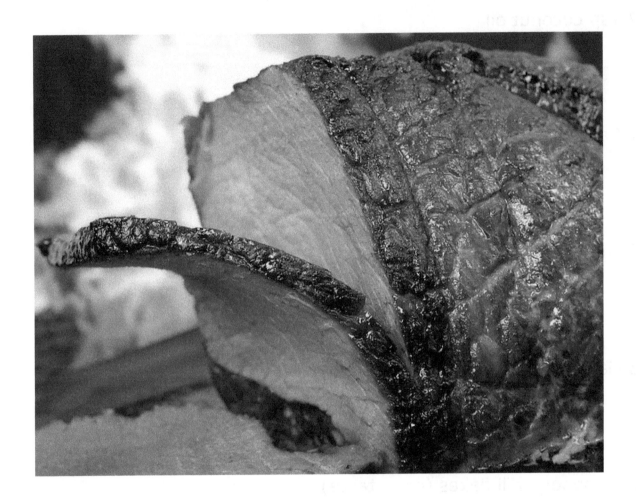

Incredible Warming Moroccan spices create this balanced tagine perfect for cold autumn and chilly evenings. Drink buckwheat to get an excess overall health kick!

Ingredients

2 Tsp coconut oil

1 Red onion, chopped

2cm ginger, grated

3 Garlic cloves, crushed or grated

1 teaspoon chili flakes (or to taste)

2 Tsp cumin seeds

1 cinnamon stick

2 teaspoons ground turmeric

800g lamb neck fillet, cut into 2cm chunks

1/2 Tsp salt

100g Medjool dates, pitted and sliced

400g Tin chopped berries, and half of a can of plain water

500g Butternut squash, chopped into 1cm cubes

400g Tin chickpeas, drained

2 Tsp fresh coriander (and extra for garnish)

Buckwheat, Cous-cous, flatbread or rice to function

Method

1. Pre Heat Your oven to 140C.

2. Drizzle Roughly 2 tbsp of coconut oil into a large ovenproof saucepan or cast-iron casserole dish. Add the chopped onion and cook on a gentle heat, with the lid for around five minutes, until the onions are softened but not too brown.

3. Insert The grated ginger and garlic, chili, cumin, cinnamon, and garlic. Stir well and cook 1 minute with off the lid. Add a dash of water when it becomes too humid.

4. Next, add from the lamb balls. Stir to coat the beef from the spices and onions, then add the salt chopped meats and berries and roughly half of a can of plain water (100-200ml).

5. Bring The tagine into the boil and put the lid and put on your skillet for about 1 hour and fifteen minutes.

6. Ten Moments prior to the conclusion of this cooking period, add the chopped butternut squash and drained chickpeas. Stir everything together, place the lid back and go back to the oven to the last half an hour of cooking.

7. When That, the tagine is able to remove from the oven and then stir fry throughout the chopped coriander. Drink buckwheat, couscous, flatbread, or basmati rice.

Notes

In case You really do not have an ovenproof saucepan or cast iron casserole dish, then only cook the tagine at a standard saucepan until it must go from the oven and transfer the tagine to a routine lidded skillet before placing in the oven. Add in an additional five minutes of cooking time and energy to allow the simple fact that the noodle dish will probably be needing additional time to warm up.

Prawn Arrabbiata-Sirtfood Recipes

Ingredients

125-150 G Beef or cooked prawns (Ideally king prawns)

65 Gram Buckwheat pasta

1 Tablespoon Extra virgin coconut oil

To get the arrabbiata sauce

40 G Red onion, finely chopped

1 Garlic clove, finely chopped

30 Gram celery, thinly sliced

1 Bird's eye chili, finely chopped

1 Tsp Dried mixed veggies

1 Tsp extra-virgin coconut oil

2 Tablespoon White wine (optional)

400 Gram Tinned chopped berries

1 tbsp Chopped parsley

Method

1. Fry the garlic, onion, celery, and peppermint and peppermint blossoms at the oil over moderate-low heat for 1--2 weeks. Turn up the heat to medium, bring the wine and cook 1 second. Add the berries and leave the sauce simmer over moderate-low heat for 20--half an hour, until it's a great rich texture. In the event you're feeling that the sauce is becoming too thick, simply put in just a very little water.

2. As the sauce is cooking, attract a bowl of water to the boil and then cook the pasta as per the package directions. Once cooked to your dish, drain, then toss with the olive oil and also maintain at the pan before needed.

3. If you're utilizing raw prawns, put them into your sauce and cook for a further 3--four minutes, till they've turned opaque and pink, then add the parsley and function. If you're using cooked prawns, insert them using the skillet, then bring the sauce to the boil and then function.

4. Add the cooked pasta into the sauce, then mix thoroughly but lightly and function.

Turmeric Baked Salmon-Sirtfood Recipes

Ingredients

125-150 Gram Skinned Salmon

1 Tsp extra-virgin coconut oil

1 Tsp Ground turmeric

1/4 Juice of a lemon

To get The hot celery

1 Tsp extra-virgin coconut oil

40 G Red onion, finely chopped

60 Gram Tinned green peas

1 Garlic clove, finely chopped

1 Cm fresh ginger, finely chopped

1 Bird's eye chili, finely chopped

150 Gram Celery, cut into 2cm lengths

1 Tsp darkened curry powder

130 Gram Tomato, cut into 8 wedges

100 Ml vegetable or pasta stock

1 tbsp Chopped parsley

Method

Heat the oven to 200C / gas mark 6.

Start using the hot celery. Heat a skillet over moderate-low heat, then add the olive oil, then the garlic, onion, ginger, celery, and peppermint. Fry lightly for two-three minutes until softened but not colored, you can add the curry powder and cook for a further minute.

Insert the berries afterward, your lentils and stock, and simmer for 10 seconds. You might choose to increase or reduce the cooking time according to how crunchy you'd like your own sausage.

Meanwhile, mix the garlic olive oil and lemon juice and then rub the salmon. # Set on the baking dish and cook 8--10 seconds.

In order to complete, stir the skillet throughout the celery and function with the salmon.

Coronation Steak Salad-Sirtfood Recipes

Ingredients

75 G Natural yogurt

Juice Of 1/4 of a lemon

1 Tsp Coriander, sliced

1 Tsp Ground turmeric

1/2 Tsp darkened curry powder

100 G Cooked chicken , cut to bite-sized pieces

6 Walnut halves, finely chopped

1 Medjool date, finely chopped

20 G Crimson pumpkin, diced

1 Bird's eye illuminates

40 Gram Rocket, to function

Method

Mix The lemon, carrot juice, spices, and coriander together in a bowl. Add all of the remaining **Ingredients** and serve on a bed of this rocket.

Baked Potatoes With Spicy Chickpea Stew-Sirtfood Recipes

Kind Of Mexican fauna matches North African Taginethis Spicy Chickpea Stew is very flavorful and also makes an excellent topping for baked potatoes, also it simply appears to be vegan, vegetarian, gluten-free and dairy-free. Plus, it comprises chocolate.

Ingredients

4 6 Celery, pricked all over

2 Tsp coconut oil

2 Red onions, finely chopped

4 Cloves garlic, crushed or grated

2cm ginger, grated

1/2 -2 teaspoons chili flakes (depending on how hot you enjoy stuff)

2 tablespoons cumin seeds

2 Tsp turmeric

Splash Of water

2 x 400g tins chopped tomatoes

2 Tablespoons unsweetened cocoa powder (or even cacao)

2 X 400g tins chickpeas (or kidney beans if you would like) including the chick-pea water do not DRAIN!!

2 Yellow peppers (or any color you would like!) , chopped into bitesize pieces

2 Tablespoons parsley and extra for garnish

Salt And pepper to taste

Negative Salad

Method

1. Pre Heat The oven to 200C, however, you are able to prepare all of your own **Ingredients**.

2. When The oven is still hot enough to set your lemon potatoes from the oven and cook for 1 hour or so until they do the way you prefer them.

3. Once The potatoes come from the oven, then place the coconut oil and sliced red onion into a large wide saucepan and cook lightly, with the lid for five minutes until the onions are tender but not brown.

4. Remove The lid and then add the ginger, garlic, cumin, and simmer. Cook for a further minute on very low heat, then add the garlic and a tiny dab of water and then cook for another moment, just take care never to allow the pan to get too tender.

5. Next, Add from the berries, cocoa powder (or even cacao), chickpeas (including the chickpea water) and salt. Bring to the boil, and then simmer on a very low heat for 4-5 seconds before the sauce is thick and unctuous (but do not allow it to burn up) . The

stew ought to be performed at exactly the exact same period as the legumes.

6. Finally, Stir at the two tbsp of parsley, plus a few pepper and salt if you desire, and also serve the stew in addition to the chopped sausage, possibly with a very simple salad.

Kale And Red Onion Dhal With Buckwheat-Sirtfood Recipes

Delicious And very wholesome, this Kale and Red Onion Dhal using Buckwheat are quick and simple to generate and naturally gluten-free, dairy-free, vegetarian, and vegetarian.

INGREDIENTS

1 Tbsp coconut oil

1 Small red onion, chopped

3 Garlic cloves, crushed or grated

2 Cm lemon, grated

1 Birdseye chili, deseeded and finely chopped (more if you like things sexy!)

2 Tsp turmeric

2 teaspoons garam masala

160g Red lentils

400ml Coconut milk

200ml Water

100g Kale (or lettuce are a terrific alternative)

160g buckwheat (or brown rice)

METHOD

1. Put The coconut oil in a large, deep saucepan and then add the chopped onion. Cook on very low heat, with the lid for five minutes until softened.

2. Insert The ginger, garlic, and chili and cook 1 minute.

3. Insert The garlic, garam masala, and a dash of water and then cook for 1 minute.

4. Insert The reddish peas, coconut milk, and also 200ml water (try so only by half filling the coconut milk could with water and stirring it in the saucepan).

5. Mix Everything together thoroughly and then cook for 20 minutes over a lightly heat with the lid . Stir occasionally and add just a little bit more water in case the dhal starts to stand.

6. Later 20 seconds add the carrot, stir thoroughly and then replace the lid, then cook for a further five minutes (1 2 minutes if you are using spinach)

7. Around 1-5 minutes ahead of the curry is ready, set the buckwheat at a medium saucepan, and then put in lots of warm water. Bring back the water to the boil and then cook for 10 minutes (or only a little longer in case you would rather your buckwheat softer. Drain the buckwheat at a sieve and function with the dhal.

Char-grilled Steak Having A Dark Wine Jus, Onion Rings, Garlic Kale, And Herb Roasted Potatoes

INGREDIENTS:

100g potatoes, peeled and cut into 2cm dice

1 Tbsp extra virgin coconut oil

5g parsley, finely chopped

50g Red onion, chopped into circles

50g Lettuce, chopped

1 garlic clove, finely chopped

120--150g X-ray 3.5cm-thick beef noodle beef or 2cm-thick sirloin beef

40ml Red wine

150ml Beef inventory

1 Tsp tomato purée

1 Tsp cornflour, dissolved in 1 tablespoon water

Guidelines:

Heating The oven to 220ºC/gas .

Put The sausage in a saucepan of boiling water, then return to the boil and then cook 4minutes, then empty. Put in a skillet with 1 tbsp of the oil and then roast in the oven for 3-5 --4-5 minutes. Twist the berries every 10 minutes to ensure even cooking. After cooked remove from the oven, sprinkle with the chopped parsley and mix well.

Fry The onion 1 tsp of the oil over a moderate heat for 5 minutes -1 minute, until tender and well caramelized. Maintain heat. Steam the kale for two-three minutes . Stir the garlic lightly in 1/2 tsp of oil for 1 minute, until tender but not colored. Insert the spinach and simmer for a further 1--two minutes, until tender. Maintain heat.

Heating An ovenproof skillet on high heat until smoking. Lay the beef from 1/2 a tsp of the oil and then fry from the skillet over a moderate-highgh temperature in accordance with just how you would like your beef done.If you prefer your beef moderate, it'd be wise to sear the beef and also transfer the pan into a toaster place in 220ºC/petrol 7 and then finish the cooking which manner to your prescribed occasions.

Remove The meat from the pan and put aside to break. Add your wine into the skillet to bring any meat up residue. Bubble to decrease the wine by half an hour until syrupy, along with a flavor that is concentrated.

Insert The inventory and tomato purée into the beef pan and bring to the boil, add the cornflour paste to thicken your sauce, then adding it only a little at a time till you've got your preferred consistency. Stir in just about anyone of those juices out of the dinner that is rested and serve with the roasted lettuce, celery, onion rings, and red berry sauce.

Kale And Black-currant Smoothie

2 Tsp honey

1 Cup freshly made green-tea

10 Infant spinach leaves stalk removed

1 Ripe banana

40 Gram blackcurrants washed and stalk removed

6 Ice cubes

Stir The honey to the green tea before dissolved. Whiz each of the **Ingredients** together in a blender until smooth. Drink instantly.

DINNER RECIPES

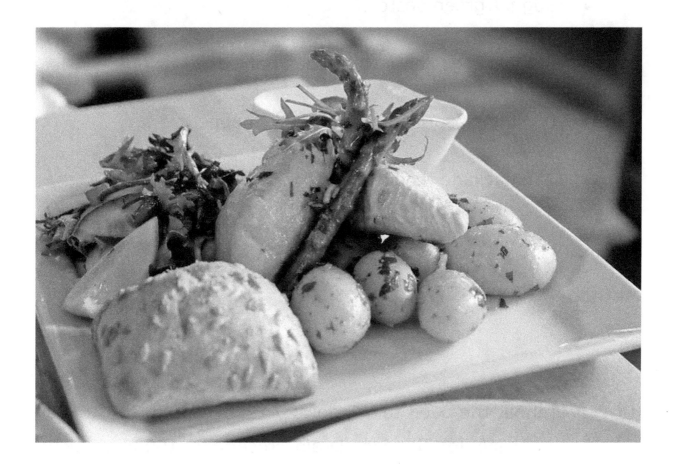

Pesto salmon pasta noodles recipe

Ingredients

- 350g penne

- 2 x 212g tins cherry salmon, drained

- 1 lemon, zested and juiced

- 190g jar green pesto

- 250g package cherry tomatoes halved

- 100g bunch spring onions, finely chopped

- 125g package reduced-fat mozzarella

Method

1. Preheat the oven to Windows 7, 220°C, buff 200°C. Boil the pasta for 5 mins. Drain, reserving 100ml drinking water.

2. Meanwhile, at a 2ltr ovenproof dish, then mix the salmon, lemon zest, and juice, then pesto (booking 2 tablespoons)berries and half of the spring onions; season.

3. Mix the pasta and reserved cooking water to the dish. Mix the allowed pesto using 1 tablespoon water and then drizzle on the pasta. Gently within the mozzarella, top with

the rest of the spring onions and bake for 25 mins until golden.

Sri Lankan-style sweet potato curry recipe

Ingredients

- 1/2 onion, roughly sliced

- 3 garlic cloves, roughly sliced

- 25g sliced ginger, chopped and peeled

- 15g fresh coriander stalks and leaves split leaves sliced

- two 1/2 tablespoon moderate tikka curry powder

- 60g package cashew nuts

- 1 tablespoon olive oil

- 500g Redmere Farms sweet potatoes, peeled and cut into 3cm balls

- 400ml tin Isle Sun Coconut-milk

- 1/2 vegetable stock block, created as much as 300ml

- 200g Grower's Harvest long-grain rice

- 300g frozen green beans

- 150g Redmere Farms lettuce

- 1 Suntrail Farms lemon, 1/2 juiced, 1/2 cut into wedges to function

Method

1. Set the onion, ginger, garlic, coriander stalks, tikka powder along with half of the cashew nuts in a food processor. Insert 2 tablespoons water and blitz to a chunky paste.

2. At a large skillet, warm the oil over moderate heat. Insert the paste and cook, stirring for 5 mins. Bring the sweet potatoes, stir, then pour into the coconut milk and stock. Bring to the simmer and boil for 25-35 mins before the sweet potatoes are tender.

3. Meanwhile, cook the rice pack directions. Toast the rest of the cashews at a dry skillet.

4. Sti-R the beans into the curry and then simmer for two mins. Insert the lettuce in handfuls, allowing each to simmer before adding the following; simmer for 1 minute. Bring the lemon juice, to taste, & the majority of the coriander leaves. Scatter on the remaining coriander and cashews, then use the rice and lemon wedges.

Chicken liver along with tomato ragu recipe

Ingredients

- 2 tablespoon olive oil

- 1 onion, finely chopped

- 2 carrots, scrubbed and simmer

- 4 garlic cloves, finely chopped

- 1/4 x 30g pack fresh ginger, stalks finely chopped, leaves ripped

- 380g package poultry livers, finely chopped, and almost any sinew removed and lost

- 400g tin Grower's Harvest chopped berries

- 1 chicken stock cube, created around 300ml

- 1/2 tsp caster sugar

- 300g penne

- 1/4 Suntrail Farms lemon, juiced

Method

1. Heat 1 tablespoon oil in a large skillet, over a low-medium heating system. Fry the onion and carrots to 10 mins, stirring periodically. Stir in the ginger and garlic pops and cook 2 mins more. Transfer into a bowl set aside.

2. Twist the pan into high heat and then add the oil. Bring the chicken livers and simmer for 5 mins until browned. Pour the onion mix to the pan and then stir in the tomatoes, sugar, and stock. Season, bring to the boil, and then simmer for 20 mins until reduced and thickened, and also the liver is cooked through. Meanwhile, cook pasta to package guidelines.

3. Taste the ragu and put in a second pinch of sugar more seasoning, if needed. Put in a squeeze of lemon juice to taste and stir in two of the ripped basil leaves. Divide the

pasta between four bowls, then spoon across the ragu and top with the rest of the basil.

Minted Lamb with a couscous salad recipe

Ingredients

- 75g Cous-cous

- 1/2 chicken stock block, composed to 125ml

- 30g pack refreshing flat-leaf parsley, sliced

- 3 mint sprigs, leaves picked and sliced

- 1 tablespoon olive oil

- 200g pack suspended BBQ minted lamb leg beans, De-frosted

- 200g lettuce berries, sliced

- 1/4 tsp, sliced

- 1 spring onion, sliced

- pinch of ground cumin

- 1/2 lemon, zested and juiced

- 50g reduced-fat salad cheese

Method

1. Place the couscous into a heatproof bowl and then pour on the inventory. Cover and set aside for 10 mins, then fluff with a fork and stir in the herbs.

2. Meanwhile, rub a little oil within the lamb steaks and season. Cook to package guidelines, then slit.

3. Mix the tomatoes, cucumber and spring onion into the couscous with the oil, the cumin, and lemon juice and zest. Crumble on the salad and serve with the bunny.

Jack Fruit tortilla bowls recipe

To get A winning beef - and - dairy-free dinner idea for just two, look no farther than this particular colorful Mexican Jack fruit recipe. With barbecued legumes, corn, and brilliant veg, you are going to wish to create this simple vegetarian meal over and over. See strategy

- Serves 2

- 5 mins to prepare and 15 mins to cook

- 354 calories serving

- healthful

Ingredients

- Two Sweet Corn cobettes

- 1 red chili, finely chopped

- 2 teaspoon olive oil

- 1 lime, juiced

- 15g fresh coriander, chopped, plus extra to garnish

- 150g package stained Jack Fruit in Texmex sauce

- 210g tin kidney beans, drained

- 125g roasted red peppers (in the jar), drained and chopped

- two whitened tortilla packs

- 1/2 round lettuce, ripped

Method

- Heat a griddle Pan on a high temperature (or light a barbecue). Griddle that the cobettes to get 10 12 Mins, turning until cooked and charred throughout. Remove from the pan and also Stand upright onto a plank. Use a sharp

93

knife to carefully reduce the Span of this corn, staying near to the heart, to clear away the kernels. Mix That the kernels with the eucalyptus oil, half of the carrot juice along with half an hour of the coriander.

- Heating the Jack fruit and sauce in a saucepan with the legumes, peppers, staying lime Coriander and juice on medium-low heating for 3-4 mins until heated Through; now.

Griddle the wraps for 10 20 secs each side to char. Tear into pieces and serve together with all the Jack Fruit lettuce And sweet corn salsa.

Carrot, courgette and halloumi Hamburgers recipe

Want Some veggie beans inspiration for the next grill? This carrot, courgette, and halloumi hamburger recipe is packaged with grated veg and creates a switch from bean hamburgers. Layer up using chopped tzatziki, delicate pineapple ribbons, and salad for a simple vegetarian barbecue winner. See strategy

- Serves 4

- 20 mins to prepare and 10 mins to cook

- 523 calories serving

- wholesome

Ingredients

- 1 big carrot, grated

- 1 large courgette, grated

- 225g halloumi, grated

- 2 spring onions, finely chopped

- 90g Bread Crumbs

- 1 tablespoon ground cumin

- 1 tablespoon ground coriander

- 1/2 teaspoon salt

- 2 tbsp

- Two tablespoons flour

- 4 brioche buns, halved

- 50g baby spinach leaves

- 1 big tomato, sliced

- 1 small red onion, chopped

- 1/2 pineapple, peeled into ribbons

- tzatziki, to function

Method

1. Place the courgette into a clean tea towel and squeeze to eradicate any liquid. Hint into a big bowl and then add the carrot, halloumi, onion, bread crumbs, cumin, coriander, eggs, salt, and flour. Stir well to mix.

2. Put simply over half the mix in a food processor and pulse until the mixture starts to stay . Reunite back this into the booked mix and mix well.

3. Divide the mix into 4 and then form into patties. Heat a grill or griddle pan into a moderate heat. Cook the hamburgers for 45 mins each side until golden and cooked through.

4. Insert the hamburger buns into the grill till lightly toasted. To assemble the burgers, put lettuce leaves on the base of each bun. Top with all the hamburger, a piece of tomato, pineapple ribbon along with a spoonful of tzatziki.

Rita's 'Rowdy' enchiladas recipe

When They all remain, Rita's kiddies really are a rowdy group. But there is something that is sure to create a silent silence into the dining table, which is her chicken enchiladas. Made out of sweet red peppers, Chicken feeding, and spices wrapped up within tortilla wraps and roasted with a spicy black bean tomato sauce and grated cheese, then it is not Tough to see exactly why. View **Method**

- Serves 4

- 1-5 mins to prepare and 55 mins to cook

- 757 carbs serving

- Freezable

Ingredients

- Two large chicken breasts (about 400g)

- 2 red peppers, thinly chopped

- 1 tablespoon olive oil

- 3/4 tsp mild chili powder

- 1 teaspoon 1/2 tsp ground cumin

- 3/4 tsp smoked paprika

- 80g grated mozzarella

- 8 Plain Tortilla Wraps

- 65g ripe Cheddar, grated

- 10g fresh coriander, roughly sliced

The sauce

- 1 tablespoon olive oil

- 1/2 onion, finely chopped

- 2 tsp cloves, crushed

- 500g tomato passata

- 1 tablespoon chipotle chili paste

- 400g tin black beans drained and rinsed

- 1/2 lime, juiced

Method

1. Preheat the oven to gas 5, 190°C, buff 170°C. Set the chicken at a 20 x 30cm skillet with all the pepper olive oil, chili powder, cumin, and paprika. Mix to coat, then cover with foil. Roast for 25-30 mins before the chicken is cooked and tender with no pink meat remains. Take out the chicken from the dish and then shred with two forks. Reserve in a bowl.

2. Meanwhile, make the sauce. Heat the oil in a saucepan on a low heat and cook the garlic and onion for 10 mins. Stir from the passata and chipotle chili glue; increase heat to moderate, bring to a simmer and cook for a further 10 mins, stirring periodically. Bring the beans and carrot juice season.

3. Mix one-third of this sauce plus half of the mozzarella to the cultured broccoli and chicken.

4. To gather, spoon 4 tablespoons of this sauce in exactly the exact baking dish before. Spoon a bit of the chicken mixture down the middle of each tortilla, roll up, and then put it from the dish. Repeat with the tortillas and filling, then placing them alongside in order that they do not shatter. Pour the remaining sauce on the top and then scatter within the Cheddar and remaining mozzarella. Bake in the oven for 20-25 mins until the cheese has melted and begun to brownish. Scatter together with all the coriander to function.

Freezing And defrosting recommendations

Cook As educated and let it cool completely. Subsequently, move to an airtight, freezer-safe container, seal, and freeze up to 1-3 weeks. Guarantee the meatballs are underwater in the sauce since they are going to freeze far better. To serve, defrost thoroughly in the refrigerator overnight before reheating. To serve, put in a bowl over moderate heat, stirring occasionally until the dish is heated throughout.

Full-of-veg hash recipe

To get A simple solution to lure all of the households to eat more veg, try out this curry hash recipe together with carrots, onions, courgettes, parsley, and topped with an egg. This family preferred is created from massaging the veg, meaning there is hardly any hands-free moment; therefore, it's fantastic for rapping through to busy weeknights. See strategy

Ingredients

- 750g potatoes, pared and grated

- 2 tablespoon olive oil

- 100g streaky bacon, roughly sliced

- 2 red onions, finely chopped

- 300g carrots, peeled and diced

- two courgettes, diced

- 2 garlic cloves, crushed

- 4 eggs

- 5g refreshing flat-leaf parsley, sliced

- 1 red chili, chopped (optional)

- 1/2 x 340g jar pickled red cabbage

Method

1. Preheat the oven to Windows 7, 220°C, buff 200°C. Bring a bowl of soapy water to the boil and then simmer the potatoes for 5 mins, then drain and put aside.

2. Heat 1 tablespoon oil in a large, ovenproof skillet on a high heat and fry the bacon for 5 mins until crispy. Add the carrots, onions, courgettes, onions, and garlic; season and then cook for 5 mins. Transfer the pan into the oven and bake for 25-30 mins before the veg is tender and gold.

3. Meanwhile, heat the remaining oil into a skillet on medium-high heating and fry the eggs 2-3 mins or until cooked to your liking.

4. Split the hash between two plates and top each with lettuce. Scatter with parsley and simmer, then function with the pickled red cabbage onto both

Bacon and egg fried rice recipe

Cook This up egg and bacon fried rice for a fast and effortless d,inner. Adding streaky bacon brings extra feel and flavor for the wallet-friendly stirfry. See strategy

Ingredients

- 350g long-grain rice, well rinsed

- 1 $^1/_2$ tablespoon olive oil

- 100g streaky bacon, diced

- two peppers, finely chopped

- 2 red onions, finely chopped

- 200g carrots, peeled and coarsely grated

- 2 garlic cloves, crushed

- 5cm slice ginger, peeled and grated

- 1 red chili, finely chopped (optional)

- 2 eggs

- 2 tsp soy sauce

Method

- Cook the rice in a big bowl of warm water for 10 mins until not quite tender. Drain, rinse with warm water and drain . Setaside.

- Meanwhile, warm 1/2 tablespoon oil in a skillet on a high heat and fry the bacon for 5 7 mins until golden and crispy. Remove from the pan using a slotted spoon and place aside. Add 1 tablespoon oil and fry the peppers for 10 mins until lightly bubbling. Add the carrots, onions, ginger, garlic, and chili and fry over a moderate-high temperature for 5 mins more.

- Insert the rice and bacon and simmer for 5 mins, stirring often. Push the rice mix to a single side of this pan and then crack the eggs to the gap. Beat the eggs with a wooden spoon, then stir throughout the rice. Cook for 2 mins, then add the soy sauce and then remove from heat. Split between 4 shallow bowls to function.

Super-speedy prawn risotto

Heating 1 tablespoon coconut oil in a skillet on medium-high heat and then put in 100g Diced Onion; cook 5 mins. Insert 2 x 250g packs whole-grain Rice & Quinoa along with 175ml hot vegetable stock (or plain water), together side 200g suspended Garden Peas. Gently split using rice using a wooden spoon. Cover and cook 3 mins, stirring occasionally, you can add two x 150g packs Cooked and Peeled King Prawns. Cook for 12 mins before prawns, peas, and rice have been piping hot, and the majority of the liquid was consumed. Remove from heat. Chop 1/2 x 85g tote water-cress and stir throughout; up to taste. Top with watercress leaves and pepper to function.

Ingredients:

100g Diced Onion

Two X 250g packs whole-grain Rice & Quinoa

200g Frozen Garden Peas

Two x 150g packs Cooked and Peeled King Prawns

1/285g Tote water-cress

SNACKS & DESSERTS RECIPES

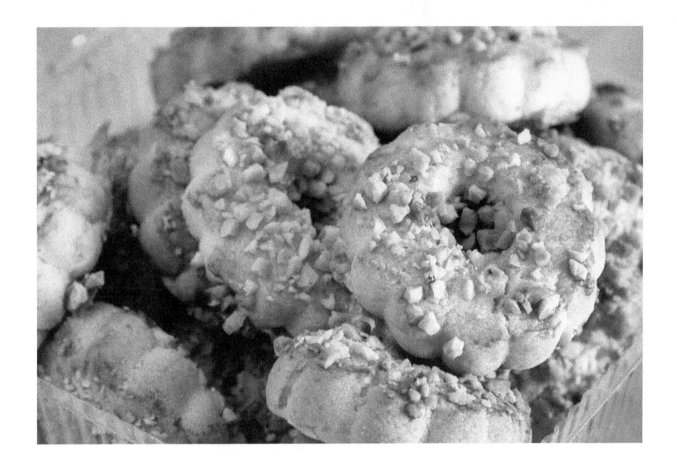

Lemon Ricotta Cookies with Lemon Glaze

Ingredients

- Two 1/2 cups all-purpose flour

- 1 tsp baking powder

- 1 tsp salt

- 1 tbsp unsalted butter softened

- 2 cups of sugar

- 2 capsules

- 1 teaspoon (15-ounce) container whole-milk ricotta cheese

- 3 tbsp lemon juice

- 1 lemon, zested

- Glaze:

- 1 1/2 cups powdered sugar

- 3 tbsp lemon juice

- 1 lemon, zested

Guidelines

1. Preheat the oven to 375 degrees F.

2. At a medium bowl, combine the flour, baking powder, and salt. Setaside.

3. From the big bowl, blend the butter and the sugar levels. With an electric mixer, beat the sugar and butter until light and fluffy, about three minutes. Add the eggs1 at a time, beating until incorporated.

4. Insert the ricotta cheese, lemon juice, and lemon zest. Beat to blend. Stir in the dry skin.

5. Line two baking sheets with parchment paper. Spoon the dough (approximately 2 tablespoons of each cookie) on the baking sheets. Bake for fifteen minutes, until slightly golden at the borders. Remove from the oven and allow the biscuits remaining baking sheet for about 20 minutes.

6. Glaze:

7. Combine the powdered sugar lemon juice and lemon peel in a small bowl and then stir until smooth. Spoon approximately 1/2-tsp on each cookie and make use of the back of the spoon to lightly disperse. Allow glaze harden

for approximately two hours. Pack the biscuits to a decorative jar.

Home-made Marshmallow Fluff

Ingredients

- 3/4 cup sugar

- 1/2 cup light corn syrup

- 1/4 cup water

- ⅛ tsp salt

- 3 little egg whites egg whites

- 1/4 tsp cream of tartar

- 1 teaspoon 1/2 tsp vanilla infusion

Guidelines

1. In a little pan, mix together sugar, corn syrup, salt, and water. Attach a candy thermometer into the side of this

pan, which makes sure it will not touch the underside of the pan. Setaside.

2. From the bowl of a stand mixer, combine egg whites and cream of tartar. Begin to whip on medium speed with the whisk attachment.

3. Meanwhile, turn the burner on top and place the pan with the sugar mix onto heat. Allow mix into a boil and heat to 240 degrees, stirring periodically.

4. The aim is to find the egg whites whipped to soft peaks and also the sugar heated to 240 degrees at near the same moment. Simply stop stirring the egg whites once they hit soft peaks.

5. Once the sugar has already reached 240 amounts, turn noodle onto reducing. Insert a little quantity of the popular sugar mix and let it mix. Insert still another little sum of the sugar mix. Carry on to add mix slowly, and that means you never scramble the egg whites.

6. After all of the sugar was added into the egg whites, then turn the rate of this mixer and also keep to overcome concoction for around 79 minutes until the fluff remains glossy and stiff. In roughly the 5 minute mark, then add vanilla extract.

7. Use fluff immediately or store in an airtight container in the fridge for around two weeks.

Guilt Totally free Banana Icecream

Ingredients

- 3 quite ripe banana - peeled and rooted

- a couple of chocolate chips

- two Tbsp skim milk

Guidelines

1. Throw all **Ingredients** into a food processor and blend until creamy.

2. Eat freeze and appreciate afterward.

Perfect Little PB Snack Balls

Ingredients

- 1/2 cup chunky peanut butter

- 3 Tbsp flax seeds

- 3 Tbsp wheat germ

- 1 Tbsp honey or agave

- 1/4 cup powder

Guidelines

1. Blend dry **Ingredients** and adding from the honey and peanut butter.

2. Mix well and roll into chunks and then conclude by rolling into wheatgerm.

Dark Chocolate Pretzel Cookies

Ingredients

- 1 cup yogurt

- 1/2 tsp baking soda

- 1/4 teaspoon salt

- 1/4 tsp cinnamon

- 4 Tbsp butter softened

- 1/3 cup brown sugar

- 1 egg

- 1/2 tsp vanilla

- 1/2 cup dark chocolate chips

- 1/2 cup pretzelstsp chopped

Guidelines

1. Pre Heat oven to 350 degrees.

2. At a medium bowl, whisk together the sugar, butter, vanilla, and egg.

3. In another bowl, stir together the flour, baking soda, and salt.

4. Stir the bread mixture in using all the moist components, along with the chocolate chips and pretzels until just blended.

5. Drop large spoonfuls of dough on an unlined baking sheet.

6. Bake for 15-17 minutes, or until the bottoms are somewhat all crispy.

7. Allow cooling on a wire rack.

Mascarpone Cheesecake with Almond Crust

Ingredients

- Crust

- 1/2 cup slivered almonds

- 8 tsp -- or 2/3 cup graham cracker crumbs

- 2 tbsp sugar

- 1 tbsp salted butter melted

- Filling

- 1 (8-ounce) packages cream cheese, room temperature

- 1 (8-ounce) container mascarpone cheese, room temperature

- 3/4 cup sugar

- 1 tsp fresh lemon juice (I needed to use imitation Lemon-juice)

- 1 tsp vanilla infusion

- 2 large eggs, room temperature

Guidelines

1. For the crust: Preheat oven to 350 degrees F.Take per 9-inch diameter around the pan (I had a throw off). Finely grind the almonds, cracker crumbs sugar in a food processor or (I used my magic bullet). Bring the butter and process until moist crumbs form.

2. Press the almond mixture on the base of the prepared pan (maybe not on the surfaces of the pan). Bake the crust until it's put and start to brown, about 1-2 minutes. Cool. Decrease the oven temperature to 325 degrees F.

3. for your filling: With an electric mixer, beat the cream cheese, mascarpone cheese, and sugar in a large bowl until smooth, occasionally scraping down the sides of the jar using a rubber spatula. Beat in the lemon juice and

vanilla. Add the eggs1 at a time, beating until combined after each addition.

4. Pour the cheese mixture on the crust from the pan. Put the pan into a big skillet or Pyrex dish Pour enough hot water to the roasting pan to come halfway up ,the sides of one's skillet. Bake until the middle of this racket goes slightly when the pan is gently shaken, about 1 hour (the dessert will get business if it's cold). Transfer the cake to a stand; trendy for 1 hour. Refrigerate before the cheesecake is cold, at least eight hours.

5. ToppingI squeezed just a small thick cream at the microwave using a busted up Lindt chocolate brown -- afterward, the got a Ziploc baggie and cut out a hole at the corner then poured the melted chocolate to the baggie and used this to decorate the cake!

Marshmallow Pop Corn Balls

Ingredients

- 2 bag of microwave popcorn

- 1 12.6 ounces. Tote M&M's

- 3 cups honey roasted peanuts

- 1 pkg. 16 ounce. Massive marshmallows

- 1 cup butter, cubed

Guidelines

1. In a bowl, blend the popcorn, peanuts and M&M's.

2. In a big pot, combine marshmallows and butter.

3. Cook medium-low warmth .

4. Insert popcorn mix, blend nicely

5. Spray muffin tins with nonstop cooking spray.

6. When cool enough to handle, spray hands together with nonstick cooking spray and then shape into chunks and put into a muffin tin to carry contour.

7. Add popsicle stick into each chunk and then let cool.

8. Wrap each person in vinyl when chilled.

Home-made Ice-cream Drumsticks

Ingredients

- Vanilla ice cream

- Two Lindt Hazel Nut chunks

- magical shell - out chocolate

- sugar levels

- nuts (I mixed crushed peppers and unsalted peanuts)

- parchment newspaper

Guidelines

- Soften ice cream and mixin topping - I had two sliced Lindt hazel nutballs.

- Fill underside of sugar with magic and nuts shell and top with ice cream.

- Wrap parchment paper round cone and then fill cone over about 1.5 inches across the cap of the cone (the newspaper can help to carry its shape).

- Shirt with magical nuts and shells.

- Freeze for about 20 minutes before the ice cream is business.

Ultimate Chocolate Chip Cookie n' Oreo Fudge Brownie Bar

Ingredients

- 1 cup (2 sticks) butter, softened

- 1 cup granulated sugar

- 3/4 cup light brown sugar

- two big egg

- 1 Tablespoon pure vanilla extract

- two 1/2 cups all-purpose flour

- 1 tsp baking soda

- 1 tsp lemon

- 2 cups (12 oz) milk chocolate chips

- 1 pkg Double Stuffed Oreos

- 1 Family-size (9×1 3) Brownie mixture

- 1/4 cup hot fudge topping

Guidelines

1. Pre Heat oven to 350 degrees F.

2. Cream the butter and sugars in a large bowl using an electric mixer at medium speed for 35 minutes.

3. Add the vanilla and eggs and mix well to thoroughly combine. In another bowl, whisk together the flour, baking soda and salt, and slowly incorporate in the mixer till the bread is simply combined.

4. Stir in chocolate chips.

5. Spread the cookie dough at the bottom of a 9×1-3 baking dish that is wrapped with wax nonstick then coated with cooking spray.

6. cloth with a coating of Oreos. Mix together brownie mix, adding an optional 1/4 cup of hot fudge directly into the mixture.

7. Twist the brownie batter within the Cookie-dough and Oreos.

8. Cover with foil and bake at 350 degrees F for half an hour.

9. Remove foil and continue baking for another 15 25 minutes.

10. Let cool before cutting on brownies might nevertheless be gooey at the midst while warm, but will also place up perfectly once chilled.

Crunchy Chocolate Chip Coconut Macadamia Nut Cookies

Ingredients

- 1 cup yogurt

- 1/2 tsp baking soda

- 1/2 tsp salt

- 1 tbsp of butter, softened

- 1 cup firmly packed brown sugar

- 1/2 cup sugar

- 1 big egg

- 1/2 cup Semi-Sweet chocolate chips

- 1/2 cup sweetened flaked coconut

- 1/2 cup coarsely chopped dry-roasted the macadamia nuts

- 1/2 cup craisins

Guidelines

1. Preheat the oven to 325°F.

2. In a little bowl, whisk together the flour, oats and baking soda, and salt then places aside.

3. On your mixer bowl, then mix together the butter/sugar/egg mix.

4. Mix from the flour/oats mix until just combined and stir into the chocolate chips, craisins, nuts, and coconut.

5. Decked outsized bits on a parchment-lined cookie sheet.

6. Bake for 1-3 minutes before biscuits are only barely golden brown.

7. Remove from the oven and then leave the cookie sheets to cool at least 10 minutes.

Peach and Blueberry Pie

Ingredients

- Peach and Blueberry Pie

- **Ingredients**1 box of noodle dough

- Filling

- 5 peaches, peeled and chopped - that I used roasted peaches

- 3 cups strawberries

- 3/4 cup sugar

- 1/4 cup bread

- juice of 1/2 lemon

- 1 egg yolk, crushed

Guidelines

1. Pre Heat oven to 400 degrees.

2. Blend dough to a 9-inch pie plate.

3. In a big bowl, combine tomatoes, sugar, bread, and lemon juice, then toss to combine. Pour into the pie plate, mounding at the center.

4. Simply take an instant disk of bread and then cut into bits, then put a pie shirt and put the dough in addition to pressing on edges .

5. Brush crust with egg wash then sprinkles with sugar.

6. Set onto a parchment paper-lined baking sheet.

7. Bake at 400 for about 20 minutes, until crust is browned at borders.

8. Turn oven down to 350, bake for another 40 minutes.

9. Remove and let sit at least 30minutes.

10. Drink Vanilla Icecream.

Pear, Cranberry and Chocolate Crisp

Ingredients

- Crumble Topping:

- 1/2 cup pasta

- 1/2 cup brown sugar

- 1 tsp cinnamon

- ⅛ tsp salt

- 3/4 cup yogurt

- 1/4 cup sliced peppers

- 1/3 cup butter, melted

- 1 teaspoon vanilla

- tsp:

- 1 tbsp brown sugar

- 3 tsp, cut into balls

- 1/4 cup dried cranberries

- 1 teaspoon lemon juice

- two handfuls of milk chocolate chips

Guidelines

1. Pre Heat oven to 375.

2. Spray a casserole dish with a butter spray.

3. Put all of the topping **Ingredients** - flour, sugar, cinnamon, salt, nuts, legumes, and dried

4. butter into a bowl and then mix. Setaside.

5. In a large bowl, combine the sugar, lemon juice, pears, and cranberries.

6. Once fully blended, move to the prepared baking dish.

7. Spread the topping evenly over the fruit.

8. Stinks for about half an hour.

9. Eliminate oven stir up - disperse chocolate chips out at the top.

10. Cook for another 10 minutes.

11. Drink ice cream.

Apricot Oatmeal Cookies

Ingredients

- 1/2 cup (1 stick) butter, softened

- 2/3 cup light brown sugar packed

- 1 egg

- 3/4 cup all-purpose flour

- 1/2 tsp baking soda

- 1/2 tsp vanilla infusion

- 1/2 tsp cinnamon

- 1/4 tsp salt

- 1 teaspoon 1/2 cups chopped oats

- 3/4 cup yolks

- 1/4 cup sliced apricots

- 1/3 cup slivered almonds

Guidelines

1. Preheat oven to 350°.

2. In a big bowl, combine with the butter, sugar, and egg until smooth.

3. In another bowl, whisk the flour, baking soda, cinnamon, and salt together.

4. Stir the dry **Ingredients** to the butter-sugar bowl.

5. Now stir in the oats, raisins, apricots, and almonds.

6. I heard on the web that in this time -- it's much better to cool with the dough (therefore your biscuits are thicker)

7. Afterward, I scooped my biscuits into some parchment-lined (easier removal and wash up) cookie sheet - around two inches apart.

8. I sliced mine for approximately ten minutes - that they were fantastic!

21 DAY MEAL-PLAN

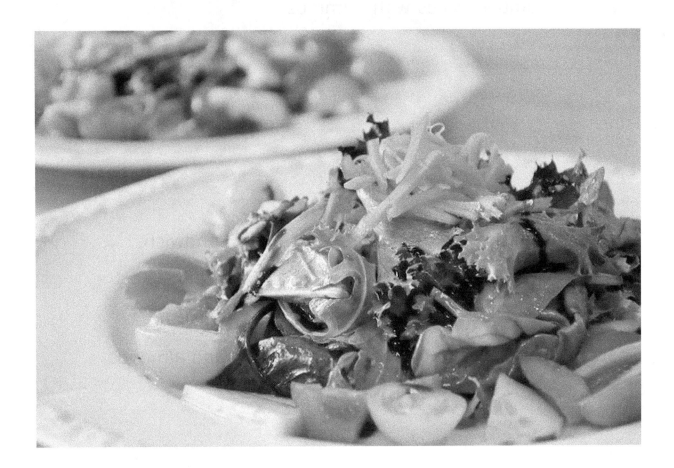

Day 1

Breakfast:

Cranberry Pecan Overnight Oats

Snack: Cucumber pieces with hummus

Lunch:

Avocado Tuna Salad or Shredded Tofu Pesto Sandwich

Snack: Apple pieces sprinkled with cinnamon and almonds

Dinner:

Left Overs: Turkey, Kale and Cauliflower Soup or Navy Bean Soup with Crispy Kale

Day 2

Breakfast:

Grain-Free Pumpkinseed Breakfast Cereal

Snack: Pear and almonds

Lunch:

Left Overs: Hearty Bean Chowder

Snack: Corn Thin Cakes with Guacamole and Fresh Salsa

Dinner:

Orange Chicken using Simple Salad OR Orange To-Fu

Day 3

Breakfast:

Sterile Eating Egg and Vegetable Basil Scramble OR Cheesy Tofu
Scramble

Snack: Celery sticks with peanut butter and raisins

Lunch:

Left-over Taco Salad or Wild Rice Burrito Bowl

Snack: Orange and also a Hard-boiled egg or couple of roasted chickpeas

Dinner:

Turkey, Kale along with Cauliflower Soup or Navy Bean Soup with Crispy Kale

Day 4

Breakfast:

Morning Meal Egg Muffins OR Chickpea Flour Omelet Muffins OR sterile Eating Peanut Buttercup Oatmeal

Snack: Banana slices with peanut butter

Lunch:

Fiesta Chicken Salad Or Easy Broccoli Salad with Almond Lemon Dressing

Snack:1/2 Cucumber with two tbsp hummus

Dinner:

Garlic Shrimp in Coconut Coffee, Tomatoes and CilantroOR Zucchini, Pea and Spinach Pesto Risotto

Day 5

Breakfast:

Protein PancakesOR Paleo Vegan Pancakes

Snack: Pear and pistachios

Lunch:

Orange Almond Salad using Avocadoor Fall Harvest Salad with Pomegranate VinaigretteSnack: Skinny Pop popcorn along with Hard-Boiled egg

Dinner:

Seafood Zucchini Pasta OR Avocado Pesto Zucchini Noodles

Day 6

Breakfast:

Left Overs: Re Heated Protein or Vegan Pancakes

Snack: Banana slices with peanut butter

Lunch:

Left Overs: Seafood Zucchini Pasta or Avocado Pesto Zucchini Noodles

Snack: Baby carrots along with guacamole

Dinner:

Sterile Eating Hearty Bean Chowder

Day 7

Breakfast:

Left-over Egg or Chick-pea Muffins OR sterile Eating Peanut Buttercup Oatmeal

Snack: Apple with Sun-flower seed/pumpkin seed course combination

Lunch:

Left-over Garlic Shrimp in Coconut Milk, Tomatoes and Cilantro OR Left-over Zucchini, Pea and Spinach Pesto Risotto

Snack: Celery sticks with guacamole

Dinner:

Taco Salad or Wild Rice Burrito Bowl with Cilantro Lime Avocado Dressing

Day 8

Breakfast:

5-Minutes Flourless Chocolate Banana Zucchini Muffins OR Pumpkin Blueberry Muffins

Snack: Brown rice salad, peanut butter, and a spoonful of honey or maple syrup

Lunch;

Left-over Orange poultry and salad or Orange To-Fu

Snack: Baby tomatoes tossed with black beans and avocado

Dinner:

Blackened Steak with Mango Avocado Salsa OR Smoky Tempeh using Fresh Peach and Cherry Tomato Salsa

Day 9

Breakfast:

Blueberry Pistachio Apple Sandwiches

Snack: 5-Minutes Flourless Chocolate Banana Zucchini Muffins

Lunch

Left-over Grilled Salmon with Mango Salsa or Smoky Tempeh

Snack: Corn Thins along with Guacamole

Dinner:

Jalapeno Turkey Burgers OR Spicy Vegan Portobello Mushroom Burgers

Day 10

Breakfast:

Morning Meal Egg Muffins OR Crust not as Sun-Dried Tomato Quiche

Snack: Baked sweet potato with peanut butter, banana, and cinnamon

Lunch

Cauliflower Mush Room Bowls

Snack: Roasted Chickpeas and berries

Dinner:

Left-over Cauliflower Mushroom Bowl using Jalapeno Turkey Burgers or Spicy Vegan Portobello Mushroom Burger

Day 11

Breakfast:

Blueberry Pistachio Apple Sandwiches

Snack: Raspberries and pistachios

Lunch

Avocado Chicken Waldorf SaladOR Vegan Waldorf Salad

Snack: Left-over cherry egg yolks or vegan egg yolks

Dinner:

Sweet Potato Noodles with Almond Dijon Vinaigrette

Day 12

Breakfast:

Left-over Breakfast egg yolks or vegan egg yolks

Snack: Banana pieces with vanilla butter and dusted with cocoa powder Lunch: Leftover sweet potato noodles

Lunch: Baby carrots and hummus

Dinner: Shrimp and Asparagus Sir FryOR Sweet and Sour Tofu

Day 13

Breakfast:

Sweet Potato Toast

Snack: 1 Larabar

Lunch: Avocado and shrimp salad (utilizing leftover beans)or sweet-sour and sweet tofu

Snack: Skinny Pop popcorn along with Hardboiled egg or couple of roasted Chickpeas

Dinner: Roasted Garlic and Herb Cod OR Easy Roasted Veggie Pizza Bites

Day 14

Breakfast:

Sweet Potato Toast

Snack: Cucumber pieces and hummus

Lunch: Leftover roasted herb and garlic codSnack: Larabar

Dinner:

Sheet Pan Chili Lime Shrimp Fajitas OR One-pan Mexican Quinoa

Day 15

Breakfast:

Berries, Beef and Coconut Shreds Cereal

Snack: Dried, pitted dates along with Peanut-butter

Lunch: Citrus Chicken Strips over Spinach Salad

Snack: Hard Boiled eggs or couple roasted chickpeas and carrots with hummus

Dinner: Tomato Basil Soup

Day 16

Breakfast:

Apple Spice Overnight Oats

Snack: Brown rice with peanut butter and banana pieces

Lunch: Left-over tomato noodle soup

Snack: Raw pepper strips together with hummus and pumpkin

Dinner:

Harvest Chicken Salad OR Lentil Cucumber Salad

Day 17

Breakfast:

Left-over: Apple Spice Overnight Oats

Snack: Dried bread and dates

Lunch:

Left-over Harvest chicken salad OR lentil cucumber salad

Snack: Apple and couple roasted chickpeas

Dinner: Steak and Veggie Quinoa Casserole OR Vegan Shepard's Pie with Gravy

Day 18

Breakfast:

Fresh fruit and Rice Breakfast Pudding

Snack: Banana and pistachios

Lunch:

Greek Quinoa Salad

Snack: Chocolate Cherry Energy Bites

Dinner: Left Overs: Chicken and Veggie Quinoa Casserole

Day 19

Breakfast:

Black Bean Scramble OR Spiced Chickpea Breakfast Scramble

Snack: Chocolate Cherry Energy Bites

Lunch:

Left Overs: Green Quinoa Salad

Snack: 100 percent apple chips and walnuts

Dinner:

Home-made Chicken Noodle SouporCurried Lentil Butternut Squash Soup

Day 20

Breakfast:

Banana Oat Protein Muffins

Snack: Apple chips dipped in peanut butter

Lunch:

Left-over Homemade Chicken Noodle Soup or Curried Butternut Squash Soup

Snack: Chocolate Cherry Energy Bites

Dinner: Steak Fajita Nachos(I propose having"Mary's Gone Crackers" rather than creating homemade bread):

Day 21

Breakfast:

Left-over Banana oat protein muffins Snack: Chewy Lemon Oatmeal Bites

Lunch: Cashew Tuna Salad Cucumber Bites(utilize a vegan mayo) OR Simple Chickpea Salad with Tomato

Snack: Baby tomatoes and pineapple pieces tossed in olive oil, balsamic vinegar plus a pinch of pepper

Dinner:

Create Ahead Grilled Chicken and Veggie Bowls(makes 8 servings to get for your week) or Chick-pea Taco BuddhaBowl

Conclusion

Here we are at the end of this little journey into the world of sirtfood taste and flavor.

Have you cooked for the whole family?

Have you practiced and practiced trying and trying again these delicious dishes?

I'm sure you have, and I'm sure you have the desire to keep discovering new recipes, so don't miss my upcoming book releases.

Obviously I advise everyone, before doing any diet, to always talk to a specialized doctor and get the best follow up, so that you can always experience rich and tasty dishes.

Thank you very much and enjoy

CPSIA information can be obtained
at www.ICGtesting.com
Printed in the USA
BVHW061230180321
602887BV00006B/766